Ketogenic Diet

A simple approach to long-term weight loss for beginners

Dr. Cynthia S. Garrett

Additionally, the information in the following pages is intended only for informational purposes and should thus be thought of as universal. As befitting its nature, it is presented without assurance regarding its prolonged validity or interim quality. Trademarks that are mentioned are done without written consent and can in no way be considered an endorsement from the trademark holder.

Table of Contents

Introduction

Congratulations on downloading this book and thank you for doing so.

The following chapters will discuss the ketogenic diet in detail. You will learn how to transition to a ketone diet, the foods you should eat, how to treat and prevent the common side effects of the ketogenic diet, and more.

There are plenty of books on this subject on the market, thanks again for choosing this one! Every effort was made to ensure it is full of as much useful information as possible.

NOTE: Consult with your healthcare provider about dietary changes and exercise that is best for your and your personal condition. Always check with your healthcare provider before starting a physical activity program or increasing the intensity of your current program.

Chapter 1: Ketogenic Diet

The ketogenic diet is known for being a very low-carb, high-fat diet. This triggers the body to create ketones which can be used as a source of energy. A ketogenic diet is known by many names such as: low carb diet, low carb high-fat diet, ketone diet, or simply keto diet; but they all follow the same concept whereby a person's caloric intake is cut down to a minimum to trigger a state known as ketosis.

A low carb diet is important to prevent your body from creating too much glucose. Glucose is the simplest energy source for the body to tap into. Insulin breaks down the glucose and takes it around the body. When this happens, the body consumes the glucose and stores fats, which is not good especially if you want to lose weight. In a ketogenic diet, the body runs on its fat reserves. Therefore, it turns the body into a fat-burning machine.

Ketogenesis

Ketogenesis is the biochemical process by which the body produces substances known as ketones or ketone bodies. Ketones are caused by the breakdown of fatty acids, as well as ketogenic amino acids in the liver.

Weight loss

The ketone diet is very famous for losing weight. It has been used by athletes and celebrities worldwide. When the body is subjected to a low-carb diet, it reaches a state known as ketosis. During ketosis, the body releases ketones as fats breakdown in the liver. This makes the ketone diet ideal for any weight loss goal. Once the body has depleted its carbs, it taps its fat reserves in order to survive. Meaning, your body turns into a fat-burning machine, which is the best state for losing weight.

Ketosis vs. ketoacidosis

Ketosis is a controlled process whereby insulin is regulated and the body is compelled to release ketones, while ketoacidosis is uncontrolled and displays a very low insulin level or a lack of it, which causes a dramatic increase in blood sugar and abnormal production of ketones. This is unhealthy and dangerous.

Why does the ketogenic diet work?

The ketogenic diet is like other diet programs: It limits the amount of calories that you consume, which causes a caloric deficit where the body uses more energy than it receives. This is the basic science behind any weight loss program. And, although "a calorie is a calorie" can easily be subjected to endless debates, only a few will argue that, one way or another, caloric restriction remains to be the key to any successful diet.

Low-carbohydrate diet

When you consume a low-carbohydrate diet, you will have a metabolism that is similar to one who is fasting. With little carbohydrates, the body taps its glycogen reserves to provide glucose to the nerves, blood, and the brain cells. Once the body has used up its glycogen stores, it starts to create glucose from amino acids of protein. This process is called gluconeogenesis. It is worth noting that even though a low-carb diet may include a high amount of protein from food, the body still makes use of the protein found in body tissues.

A simple way to determine when glycogenesis has taken place is by monitoring your urine. The production of urine in the body increases when the body releases water as it breaks down glucose or protein. Low-carb diets lead to ketosis. The body creates ketones when the glucose reserves have been depleted and when the breakdown of fat is incomplete.

As a usual part of any diet, there are foods that you should avoid eating. When you follow the ketone diet, do not eat the following:

Grains – wheat, corn, rice, cereal, grits, etc.

Sugars- cane sugar, brown sugar, honey, agave, maple syrup, etc.

Fruit – apples, bananas, oranges, melons etc.

Tubers – potato, yams, etc.

Low carb, moderate protein, high fat

The foods in a keto diet are low in carb, moderate in protein, and high in fat. The diet must be low in carbohydrates so that it will be possible to reach the state of ketosis.

A ketogenic diet is moderate in protein so that you can still build and develop your muscles. Other ketone dieters take high protein while on a keto diet – and this is not advisable. Reason: The excess protein is used by the body as another source of energy or is turned into fat. Taking too much protein can make ketosis impossible to achieve or can remove you from ketosis. Therefore, only take a moderate amount of protein.

Last but not least, the keto diet is high in fat for obvious reasons. Since the keto diet turns the body into a constant fat burning machine, you need to have fat reserves that your liver can break down to create ketones.

Fat vs. ketones

It is worth noting that on a keto diet, the body is fueled by ketones. Now, you might be wondering, how come people say that a keto diet will make your body to function using its fat reserves? This, in fact, is what makes it a fat burning machine. The answer is simple: In order to produce ketones, the body uses its fat reserves. When the fats are broken down in the liver, ketones are produced. The ketones are the end product of the breakdown of fats in the liver. However, before the body uses its fat reserves, it first gets its energy from carbs. This is the reason why the ketone diet is low in carbohydrates, because the carbs must first be depleted before the body can tap its fat reserves and turn them into ketones.

Benefits of eating moderate protein

Protein is an essential part of the keto diet. It is consists of amino acids, which build muscles. Moreover, a moderate amount of protein in your diet will not just help you build muscles; it can also help you with weight loss. Protein is very sating and will help you feel less hungry. Studies also show that protein increase energy expenditure. Although this does not offer a significant metabolic advantage, it can be considered helpful in the long run. And since protein will help you build more muscle mass, you will be constantly burning more calories, even at rest. On the negative side, too much protein can make you gain weight and kick you off of ketosis. Therefore, the keto diet strongly advises that you only take a moderate amount of protein. Protein also tends to increase your insulin level. However, if you are on a ketone diet, this would not be a problem since the ketogenic diet will compensate the said increase of insulin.

How much is a moderate amount of protein?

The amount of protein that the body needs may vary from one person to another. You can get the minimum and maximum amount of protein that you need (in grams) by multiplying your weight (in pounds) by 0.6 (minimum) and 1.0 (maximum). Be it noted that athletes and those engaged in strenuous physical activities will require a higher amount of protein. Other factors that can affect your minimum and maximum protein counts are your age, sex, amount of muscle that you already have, as well as the physical activities that you engage in.

How to measure ketosis

Ketosis is the natural state where the body relies on its fat reserves to fuel itself. However, it must be understood that ketosis is divided into different levels:

Nutritional ketosis

Ketosis only begins when your blood ketones reach 0.5 mmol/l. This means that even if you reach a point where the body begins to release ketones, it is not yet considered a state of ketosis until and unless the number of ketones reaches 0.5 mmol/l. But do not be discouraged; once the body starts producing ketones, it means that you are getting close to reaching the state of ketosis. So, just stick to your diet plan, and your body will soon be a fat burning machine.

Optimal ketone zone

As the name already implies, this is the level of ketosis that you should aim for. Optimal ketosis zone is where your ketone count reaches 1.5 − 3 mmol/l. This is the level where the body turns into a full blown burning machine, continuously burning fats at the highest rate. This is also the zone where you will experience maximum performance gains both physically and mentally.

Take note that a value of 1.7 or 2.5 or any other number has the same effect provided you remain within the said zone (1.5 – 3 mmol/l. However, the higher the value or the closer you get to 3, the closer you get to the next stage of ketosis called, starvation ketosis — which is not good.

Starvation ketosis

Starvation ketosis is when your ketone count exceeds the optimal level. The ketogenic diet is not fasting. You do not deprive yourself of food. Starvation ketosis means that your body does not get enough food, which is bad. If you ever reach this level, eat more and nourish your body.

Ketoacidosis

This is a terrible stage. The good news is that you would not reach this stage if you follow a keto diet correctly. However, if you still reach this level despite following a keto diet, it only means that something is seriously wrong. People who reach this level are usually those who suffer from type 1 diabetes with a serious lack of insulin.

Measure your level of ketosis

In order to measure your level of ketosis, you have to measure your ketones:

Blood ketone meters

Using a blood ketone meter is said to be the most reliable and accurate method to measure your level of ketosis. However, this device is a little expensive. You can purchase a good blood ketone meter for $100. The package usually comes with about 10 free test strips. These test strips are non-reusable. You can buy new test strips for about $3 – 5$ each.

Urine strips

This is the cheapest way to measure your level of ketosis. You simply have to dip a strip in your urine, wait for a few seconds, and then the color will change. The color that you get will signify your level of ketones. A dark color usually represents that you are in ketosis. It is worth noting, however, that this method is not completely reliable. The result can be unduly affected by the amount of fluids that you have taken. Moreover, once the body has already adjusted to the ketone diet, urine strips can be unreliable. Therefore, this approach is only advisable for those who are just starting out on a keto diet.

Breath ketone analyzer

This is a quick and easy way to measure your level of ketosis. Unfortunately, it is not a reliable. The result can be misleading. Also, such device requires computer connection to read your ketone level. And although you can use it as much as you want, it is quite expensive at around $150.

Do you need to reach optimal ketosis?

You might be asking if reaching optimal ketosis is a must to enjoy the benefits of the ketone diet. Ideally, you should aim to reach this level, because this is the part where the body turns into a full-blown fat burning machine. However, this does not mean that you cannot enjoy the benefits of this diet if you do not reach the state of optimal ketosis. The ketone diet is very powerful and effective that even at lower levels of ketosis, you will already reap some significant benefits. But, if you want to get more benefits, if you want to experience the maximum mental and physical performance that the ketone diet offers, then reaching the optimal zone of ketosis should be your aim.

Is it safe for you?

Generally, ketone diet is safe for everyone. After all, this type of diet relies on the natural process of the body. However, if you have diabetes or high-blood pressure, there are certain adjustments you should make so you can safely go on a ketogenic diet.

If you have diabetes, then ketone diet is good for your health. Just remember that when you go on a low-carb diet, you should also significantly your intake of insulin. The decreased blood sugar level that is a natural part of the ketone diet usually means that you will have less need for medication. For example, since the ketone diet lowers the blood sugar level, you will now have to take a smaller dose of insulin; otherwise, you will run the risk of having hypoglycemia. Therefore, always remember that once you adopt this diet, you must also adjust your medication. It is best to consult your doctor about this. It is also recommended to test your blood sugar regularly when you begin a ketogenic diet, so you can monitor your blood sugar level. If your treatment for diabetes is solely diet based or simply with Metformin, then switching to any low-carb diet such as the ketone diet is safe.

How much you should lower your insulin doses when on a ketone diet is not easy to know. To be safe, consult your doctor.

If you have high-blood pressure, then going on a ketone diet would also be beneficial for you. You have to monitor your blood pressure frequently because there is a risk of getting your blood pressure so low. And like in the case of diabetes, you should adjust your medication. The ketone diet can dramatically decrease your blood pressure, so adding the effects of your current medication will make your blood pressure drop. Again, a visit to your doctor is highly recommended and is a good way to start your ketone diet.

How many carbs should you eat?

Decreasing your carb intake is the key to ketosis. But, how much carbohydrates should remain in your diet? This depends on your body type, but most people reach ketosis by limiting their net carbs per day to 20-30 grams. Most of the time, a sudden change in your diet can give you extreme difficulty to deal with. Here are a few good ways to adjust to the ketogenic diet:

High to low

If you are just about to start a ketone diet, it is safe to assume that you are not yet in ketosis. To avoid shocking your system with a drastic drop of carb intake, you can start your keto diet with 50g net carbs. Then just gradually decrease the amount of net carbs. However, although this can help you to have an easier transition, this approach will take you more time to reach the optimum level of ketosis.

Low to high

Another method is to begin with a low number of carbs and increase it gradually per week. Beginning with a low-carb count will help you reach ketosis faster. The suggested way to do this is to first drop your net carbs to 20. You will reach ketosis on the second or third day. Once you reach the state of ketosis, you can add a bit of carbs (another 5 or 10g). The good thing about this approach is that although you will face difficulty in the beginning, it can take you to the state of ketosis extremely fast, knowing that the diet will be easier after just a few days.

Of course, you can simply reduce your carb intake right away to just 30g net carbs and wait for ketosis to kick in. It is worth noting that these refer to net carbs. 30g net carbs can be about 50g total carbohydrates. Do not feel discouraged if you do not detect the presence of ketones right away. After all, weight loss occurs even before your body starts to produce any ketone body.

Reaching the state of ketosis is simple. You just need to deplete your body of carbs and glucose, so that the body can run on its fat reserves. Yes, it will be difficult in the beginning, but it is also so much easier than fasting. Also, it is be mindful that a ketogenic diet is only very challenging in the beginning. Once the body has reached the state of ketosis and has adjusted to the diet, things will be a lot easier and your body will turn into a fat-burning machine. The difficult part is only temporary, but it offers a ton of benefits.

Zero carbohydrate

Unlike fasting, the ketone diet does not totally remove carbohydrates in your diet, simply because there is no need to do so. You can still reach ketosis even when you enjoy some carbs now and then. Many dieters experience the benefits of the ketone diet at 50g of carbs per day. Also, it is worth noting that having more ketones does not mean you will burn more fats. What is important is for you to be able to identify how much carbs you need to keep your appetite satiated. Not all bodies are the same. Some may be able to reach the state of ketosis at 50g carbs per day. If you are lucky, you might be able to do the same even with a diet of 55g daily carbs. You should also take into consideration the amount of physical activity that you engage in. if you do strenuous exercises such as running or swimming, there is a good chance that you can hit ketosis even with a slightly higher daily carb count.

Chapter 2: Benefits

Proper planning is important in starting a keto diet. This means that you will have to come up with a viable diet plan to stick to. How fast you will reach a ketogenic state depends on the foods that will compose your diet, as well as the amount of foods that you eat. Remember: the fewer carbohydrates you take, the faster you will enter ketosis.

The keto diet offers a ton of benefits from weight loss to improving mental focus and physical performance, among others. It will not only make you healthier, it will also make you feel good about your body and boost your self-esteem.

Weight loss

Weight loss is a common effect of a ketogenic diet. When a person reaches the state of ketosis, the body burns fat in the liver and produces ketones. This turns the body into an active and effective fat burning machine, where it taps and burns its fat reserves to produce ketones as fuel for the body.

Improved mental focus

Increased focus and concentration is one of the common effects of a ketone diet. When you reach the state of ketosis, the brain receives and uses a constant flow of ketones. In fact, many people, even those who are already physically fit, still rely on the ketone diet in order to improve their mental performance. Moreover, this diet avoids dramatic fluctuations of blood sugar levels.

Interestingly, many people still think that proper brain functions require lots of carbohydrates. However, this is only true if ketones are not available.

After about a week of adapting to a ketogenic diet, the brain and the body can function easily on ketones. However, it is worth noting that before you reach this stage, you will first have to face the usual challenges that accompany most low-carb diets, such as headache, mood swings, and difficulty in concentrating. Once you pass the initial stages of hardship, you can enjoy higher energy levels, as well as better mental focus.

Increased physical endurance

Since a ketone diet will allow you to have access to all the energy of your fat reserves, it can significantly develop your physical endurance.

The body's storage of carbohydrates (glycogen) can only last for a few hours of physical activity, even less. But, your fat reserves have enough energy to last for weeks, even months.

Since most people these days are used to tapping their storage of carbohydrates as a source of energy, their fat reserves are not easily available, not even to fuel their brain. This results in having a need to eat before, during, and after a workout, or even just to avoid hunger and fuel your day to day activities. The ketogenic diet solves this problem by allowing you to tap your fat reserves to fuel not only your body but also your brain. And, unlike other diets that are only good for a month or two, the state of ketosis can last forever.

The ketone diet assures you that whether you are going to compete in a competition that requires top-notch physical condition or simply want to develop your physical and mental performance, your body has more than enough energy to keep you going.

Metabolic syndrome

Various studies reveal that low-carb diets such as the ketone diet improve markers of metabolic syndrome, which include blood and insulin levels, LDL particle size, HDL cholesterol, as well as blood sugar levels, among others.

Metabolic syndrome is a term used to describe a group of risk factors that increases your risk for heart disease and other health problems, such as diabetes and stroke. While "metabolic" refers to biochemical processes involved in the normal body function, there are associated risk factors that increase your chance of developing a disease.

Metabolic Risk Factors

There are five conditions below which are considered metabolic risk factors. You can have any one of these risk factors by itself, but they tend to occur together. When three or more are present, a diagnosis of metabolic syndrome can me made.

- **A large waistline**
  Waist Circumference
  Men greater than 40 inches
  Women greater than 35 inches

- **Elevated triglyceride level**
  Triglycerides are a type of fat found in the blood.
  Equal to or grater than 150mg/dl

- **Low HDL cholesterol**
  Men less than 40 mg.dl
  Women less than 50 mg/dl
  HDL also referred to as "good" cholesterol. This is because it helps remove cholesterol from your arteries. A low HDL level increases your risk for heart disease.

- **Elevated blood pressure**
  Blood pressure is the force of blood pushing against the walls of your arteries as your heart pumps blood. If this pressure rises and remains high over time, it can damage your heart and lead to plaque buildup.

- Elevated fasting blood sugar (or you're on medicine to treat high blood sugar).

Say no to starvation

Unlike fasting, keto does not totally prohibit you from eating. In fact, it encourages you to eat a diet that is very low in carbohydrates, moderate in protein, and high in fat. Fat is satisfying and will keep you feeling "full" for a longer period than carbohydrates.

Improved triglyceride and cholesterol levels

A ketogenic diet can help improve your triglyceride and cholesterol levels. A diet that is very low on carbohydrates and high in fats can significantly increase your high-density lipoprotein cholesterol (HDL) and decrease your low-density lipoprotein cholesterol (LDL). HDL is commonly known as good cholesterol, while LDL is also known as bad cholesterol. It is important to keep these two in a balanced and healthy level. HDL protects you from heart diseases, while LDL builds up in your arteries and can dramatically increase your chances of getting a heart disease.

Treatment for type 2 diabetes

Since the ketone diet is a low-carbohydrate diet, it is proven to be effective in reversing type 2 diabetes. The main cause of type 2 diabetes is having high blood sugar. Since this sugar comes from the carbs that you eat, it means that the less sugar you eat, the less sugar will be present in the blood which, in turn, will effectively lower your blood sugar level. A dramatic drop in blood sugar level is a natural part of the ketone diet. Always keep in mind that if you are already taking medications for type 2 diabetes, you will have to adjust the dosage once you engage in a ketone diet to avoid your blood sugar from dropping too low. This is also a good way to control type 1 diabetes.

Not a zero-carb diet

A ketone diet does not ultimately remove all carbohydrates from your diet. It merely imposes a limitation or restriction on the amount of carbs that you eat. Your carbs should come from nuts, vegetables, and dairy products. You must avoid eating any refined carbohydrates, such as starch (beans, potatoes, and legumes), wheat (bread, cereals, pasta), and fruits. Exceptions to these are berries, avocado, and star fruits, which can be taken in moderation.

Chapter 3: Dangers, Side Effects, and How to Avoid Them

Like other healthy diet programs, you can expect to face certain side effects as the body takes time to adjust to your new diet. Here are effective things you can do to lessen or avoid them:

Keto flu

Ketone dieters who transition to a fat-burning mode may experience initial side-effects, such as nausea, headache, cramps, mood swings, etc. — also known as the keto flu. Here are some things you can do to help alleviate these symptoms:

Drink water – Keep yourself hydrated by drinking more water. You can also mix in some salt and lemon. As an alternative, you can also enjoy a cup of bouillon daily.

Gradual reduction of carbs – You can prepare for a ketone diet by gradually reducing your intake of carbohydrates. A sudden drop of carb intake can shock your system, which can make you feel very uncomfortable.

When you begin a ketogenic diet, you will lose water as well as electrolytes. This happens because carbohydrates retain the water and salt in the body. Consequently, if you drop your carb intake, your body also experiences a decrease in water. If you happen to experience keto flu because of dehydration, drink a glass of water mixed with salt. To add more taste, squeeze in a bit of lemon.

A body that is not used to a low-carb diet will take time to adjust. The sudden removal or dramatic decrease of carbohydrates will make the brain function with a slightly low energy. This usually gives a feeling of tiredness, nausea, and can even give a bad headache. However, these are only temporary. Once the body has adjusted to the diet and to being fueled by ketones, said side effects disappear.

If you do not want to decrease your carb intake gradually and would rather get on straight with the ketone diet, be sure to hydrate yourself with enough fluid. A cup or two of bouillon daily is said to effectively minimize the uncomfortable side effects of a ketone diet.

Bad breath

Dieters who engage in a ketone diet or any low-carb diet can experience bad breath. This smell comes from acetone, which is a ketone body. The smell is usually described as something fruity or like a nail polish remover. Now, although the term fruity seems good, it is actually not; otherwise, it would not be called as bad breath. This means that your body is turning into a fat burning machine and is creating ketones to fuel the body and the brain. This odor can also be a body odor that usually reveals itself when you exercise or sweat a lot.

It is worth noting that some people do not experience these symptoms. Others who experience these temporary symptoms notice that they disappear once the body has adapted to the diet. Here are some more things to consider:

1.   Drink more water

It is usual to experience having a dry mouth when you first engage in any low-carb diet. It is also a normal part of getting into ketosis. This results in having less saliva to clean away the bacteria in your mouth, which can result in bad breath. Therefore, make sure to drink enough fluid and keep yourself hydrated. Salt is also an excellent cleansing ingredient. You can gargle with warm salt water or simply drink a cup of water mixed with salt.

2. Oral hygiene

Maintaining a good oral hygiene is important, especially when doing a keto diet. Although brushing your teeth will not get rid of the foul smell, it can help minimize it by preventing it from mixing with other unpleasant odor.

3. Breath freshener

A breath freshener can be applied instantly and can somehow mask the smell of keto lingering in your breath.

4. Give it more time

In most cases, this kind of bad breath is only temporary, so just give it more time. It usually goes away on its own once the body has adjusted to the new diet.

5. Lower the degree of ketosis

If it does not go away after a few weeks or a month, a good way to deal with it is by reducing your degree of ketosis. You can do this by eating more carbs. Usually, people can get out of ketosis by adding 50-70g of carbs — so only add a little bit. You can also combine this with intermittent fasting.

Leg cramps

Experiencing leg cramps is common when starting on a keto diet. Although leg cramps do not usually pose much of a problem, they can be an issue when they become painful. Leg cramps are caused by the loss of magnesium because of increased urination. Here are three effective ways to prevent or cure leg cramps.

Salt and water

The magical mixture of salt water can again be used to treat and prevent leg cramps. Be sure to drink enough fluid and keep yourself hydrated. This can also help you lower the loss of magnesium.

Magnesium supplement

Since leg cramps are caused by the loss of magnesium, it is only logical to treat it by taking magnesium tablets.

Eat more carbs

As a last resort, you can increase your intake of carbohydrates. Take note, however, that this will weaken the effects of your ketone diet.

High cholesterol level

There is something serious about the keto diet taking a position that encourages consumption of foods that are high in fat. Although a low-carb, high-fat diet such as the keto diet is known for improving a dieter's cholesterol profile. However, a few people may experience some troubling result. This happens when the amount of good cholesterol exceeds the normal level. Here are some things you can do to avoid this:

Lower your fat intake

Since consuming too much high fat is the cause of this problem, try to lower your fat intake, especially when you are not feeling hungry. Also, choose drinks that have lower fat content.

Intermittent fasting

Intermittent fasting is like fasting, but it is only for a short period. This is a good way to lower your cholesterol level. For example, skip your breakfast, or simply eat only a little. You do not have to do this every day.

Use unsaturated fats

Unsaturated fats can help lower your cholesterol. In addition, they can help prevent heart diseases, including stroke. They also nourish the cells of the body.

Good choices of unsaturated fats include olive oil, avocados, almonds, fatty fish, and peanut butter, among others. Remember to always take note of the carb content.

On alcoholic beverages and intoxication

It is not hard to notice that you can easily become intoxicated when you follow a ketone diet or any low-carb diet. If you are used to drinking lots of beer, once you only take low carbs, even a bottle or two of beer can make you a bit tipsy. In other words, your alcohol tolerance will significantly decrease. This is most probably due to the liver being busy creating ketones, so it could not function completely to digest the liquor. But, the reason behind this remains unclear. In any case, once you engage in a ketogenic diet, you should be ready to deal with less alcohol tolerance. This is actually a good way to be healthy.

A problem with alcoholic drinks is the amount of carbs they contain, which is not good for a keto diet. Therefore, you should choose your drink wisely. If you are a wine drinker, you can go for dry wines. Dry wines have low carbs; therefore, they are highly recommended to anyone on a low-carb diet. Avoid sweet wines, because they usually have lots of sugar.

If you are a beer drinker, choose light beers or beers that contain little carbohydrates. Do not worry that you cannot enjoy drinking beers as much as you used to, since your alcohol tolerance also decreases when you are on a ketogenic diet. Good choices are Heineken (11g carb content), Bud Light (7g carb content), Stella Artois (13g), Select 55 (1.9g), Natural Light (3.2g), Busch Light (3.2g), Coors Light (5g), and Budweiser (11g).

If you are a hard drinker, then you are in luck. Many hard drinks have little to zero carbs, such as whiskey and brandy, and even tequila shots and martinis. If you want a touch of lady's drink then Bloody Mary is a good choice with only 7g of carbs, while a glass of margarita has 8g and Cosmopolitan has 13g of carbohydrates. But then, not all drinks are prepared the same way, so be sure to check the amount of carbs of your drink (usually written on the bottle or can), or just ask the bartender. Champagne is also an excellent choice with only 1 gram of carb per serving.

Keto rash

Many dieters who first reach ketosis experience what is called as keto rash. It is an itchy feeling. This is not only uncomfortable but can also be troublesome when you sleep. There are many theories on what causes this problem. The prevailing thought is that it is due to acetone, which is a ketone body that is present in sweat. Keto rash usually goes away on its own once the body has adjusted to the ketone diet. However, should this problem persist and you want to get rid of it quickly, here are some things you can do:

Wear comfortable clothing

Use clothes that are comfortable and appropriate for the climate. Wearing less or think clothing is recommended in order to sweating.

Air conditioning

Use air conditioning or an electric fan so you will not sweat. Keto rash happens when ketones are released as you sweat followed by the drying up of the sweat on your skin. The important thing to remember is that you should avoid sweating.

Adjust your exercises program

You can choose either to choose exercise programs that will make you perspire less or simply skip exercising completely. Especially if you just want to lose weight, walking and lightweight training are good options. If you live in a place where the climate has a naturally high temperature, you can visit a nearby mall and do your walking exercise there. Just avoid buying unhealthy foods and drinks when you get hungry.

Give it more time

Many times, all you need to do is to wait it out and allow the keto rash to disappear on its own. The body simply needs to adjust and get used to the state of ketosis. Most of the time, 1 to 3 days would be enough.

Exit the state of ketosis

If all else fails, the best way is simply to consult your doctor or simply exit the state of ketosis. You can safely exit ketosis by gradually adding more carbs in your diet. It is worth noting that even though you are not in a state of ketosis, you can still continue to enjoy the benefits of a keto diet. Unfortunately, they will not be as good as when you are in a state of ketosis. If you just want to lose weight, adding around 50-100g of carbs is usually enough to exit ketosis but still good enough to make you lose weight; but do not expect losing weight as fast as when you are in a state of ketosis.

Although the ketone diet can be used for a long term, you are also free to do it for a short-term period only. Either way, there can come a time when you simply want to just completely enjoy and not follow any strict diet program. Getting out of ketosis is easy: Just gradually add carbs to your diet.

You might be wondering if you can still try to enter the state of ketosis even if you had problems with keto rash before. The suggested answer is yes because there are people who had trouble with keto rash the first time they entered ketosis but found it to be less of a problem the second time they entered ketosis. Other times, the keto rash does not even appear on the second time you enter ketosis. Therefore, if you are serious about going on a keto diet, it is best to give it another attempt, so you can really enjoy the powerful benefits of a true ketogenic diet.

Chapter 4: Keto Foods

Unlike fasting, the ketogenic diet encourages you to eat. However, you cannot just eat any kind of food. In a keto diet, you should only eat fresh foods that are low in carbs, adequate in protein, and high in fats.

Meats

Stick to meats that have a good amount of protein and low-carb contents, such as beef, fish, eggs, etc. Eat wild-caught fish and avoid farmed fish.

Vegetables

Eat leafy greens like turnips, collards, spinach, and kale. You can also eat above ground vegetables, such as broccoli, squash, cauliflower, and zucchini.

High-fat dairy

High-fat foods are a normal part of a ketone diet. Fat also makes you feel full for a longer period. Examples: high fat cream, butter, and high cheeses.

Nuts and seeds

Nuts and seeds are packed with nutrients that can help your body stay lean and healthy. Examples: macadamias, almonds, walnuts, and sunflower seeds.

Avocado and berries

You can satisfy your sweet tooth with tasty strawberries, kiwi, blackberries, and raspberries, as well as other low glycemic impact berries.

Sweeteners

Use sweeteners that have the lowest count of carbohydrates, such as Splenda, stevia, monk fruit, Sweet n Low, etc.

Other fats

Other good sources of fats that you can incorporate into your keto diet are high-fat salad dressing, coconut oil, and saturated fats.

Keep in mind that keto diet is very low in carbohydrates, moderate in protein, and high in fat. A typical ketone diet may be represented as follows:

Fats – 70%

Protein – 25%

Carbohydrates – 5%

On average, it is suggested to take between 20-30g of net carbohydrates daily for a ketone diet. However, if you want to hit ketosis quickly, you may take fewer carbs and keep your glucose levels low. If losing weight is your purpose of doing a keto diet, then it is strongly recommended that you take note of your total carbohydrates and net carbohydrates.

You might be asking, "What is a net carbohydrate?" The answer is simple: Net carbs are your total dietary carbohydrates minus the total fiber. It is a sound advice to keep your total carbs below 35g and your net carbs less than 25g, or more ideally, below 20g.

When you engage in a ketone diet or any low-carb diet, dieters face one major enemy: hunger. The uncomfortable feeling of hunger and the strong temptation of just giving up on your diet get so strong. At this point, many dieters give in and surrender, while others stay strong and soon enjoy the benefits of their diet.

When you engage in a ketone diet and find yourself hungry, you can curb your appetite by eating nuts, peanut butter, cheese, and seeds. Do not confuse your desire to eat with the need to eat.

Broccoli

Broccoli is very common in a ketone diet. It is packed with vitamins C and K, and what is more, a cup of broccoli only contains 4g net carbs. Various studies also show that those suffering from type 2 diabetes can benefit from eating broccoli because it lowers insulin resistance. Broccoli can also protect you from some types of cancer. As such, it is a staple food in a ketone diet and is very handy.

Asparagus

Asparagus is fully packed with vitamins C, A, and K. Studies also show that it can help reduce anxiety and protect brain health.

Fungi

If you are tired of boring dishes, just add in some fungi and enjoy a flavorful meal. For examples, adding baby bellas in a mushroom cauliflower risotto will give it better texture and flavor. Baby bellas are also very low in carbs, at only 1g net carb per cup.

Mushrooms

Mushrooms have excellent anti-inflammatory properties. A study shows that those who metabolic syndrome have seen significant improvements within 16 weeks.

Squash

Most types of squash have high carbohydrates, so make sure that you pick the right squash for your diet. The best and most commonly used in a ketone diet is the summer squash. Summer squash is usually used as a noodle replacement in dishes such as Zoodles.

Zucchini

A cup of zucchini only has 3g net carbs, which makes it an excellent part of your diet plan. It is also a great source of vitamin C.

Spinach

When it comes to eating green leafy vegetables, spinach tops the list among those who engage in a ketone diet. A cup of cooked spinach only contains 3g net carbs, with almost no digestible raw carbohydrates. Therefore, if you want to supercharge your lunches with salads, spinach is one of your best and healthy options. You can easily make creamed spinach. It is high in fat and a fantastic side dish to go along with your meal. Spinach does not only contain vitamins and minerals, it also protects heart health and lowers the risks of common eye diseases.

Avocado

Although technically not considered a fruit, avocado can be eaten in place of vegetables. Avocado is high in fat, which makes it one of the foods that compose a ketone diet as a fat supplement. A cup of avocado only has 3g net carbohydrates.

It is also a fantastic source of monosaturated fats which is effective in lowering bad cholesterol and triglycerides. It is also a recommended fruit vegetable when you have electrolyte issues, because it is rich in vitamin C and potassium.

Cauliflower

Commonly known as the star of dishes, cauliflower is a versatile ingredient that can be added to different kind of meals. It can be used for pizzas, wraps, casseroles, and mashed potatoes. With only 2g net carbohydrates per cup, it is not surprising that cauliflower is one of the most commonly used ingredients in many low-carbohydrate diets.

Green bell pepper

Also known as capsicum, green bell pepper has lower carbs than other kinds or colors of bell pepper. It is very nutritious and is packed with vitamin A, as well as anti-inflammatory qualities due to the carotenoids which it contains.

You may also eat yellow or red bell peppers, because they also have low carbohydrates, at only 6g net per cup, chopped.

Green beans

Included in the legume family, greens beans have fewer carbs than other legumes. They are sometimes called as snap peas. A cup of green beans only contains 6g net carbs, which makes them an excellent addition to any meal.

Green beans do not just add texture, but they also have a ton of health benefits, including brain function improvement during aging. If you want to make it more flavorful, you may combine green beans with some pecans to add crunch.

Kale and lettuce

Used in salads worldwide, kale and lettuce are an excellent low-carbohydrate option. They are also a good source of vitamins A and C and can help lower the risks of heart diseases.

Although kale is definitely more nutritious than lettuce, it also has more carbs per serving. So, be careful how much kale you consume because carbohydrates can add up fast.

Do not Eat

If you are on a ketogenic diet, you should avoid eating the following foods:

Grains

Avoid eating grains like rice, wheat, and cereals.

Sugars

Your sugar should be kept to a minimum. Therefore avoid eating candies, honey, maple syrup, even brown sugar.

Tubers

Do not eat yams, potatoes, etc.

Fruits

Avoid or at least limit your consumption of fruits like bananas, apples, melons, etc.

Quick meal ideas

Unlike other diet programs, you will never run out of meal ideas when you go on a ketogenic diet. Whether as a meal or just a way to ease hunger, the following meal ideas are excellent for anyone on a keto diet. And, what is more, these meals are easy and quick to make.

> Fry macadamia nuts in butter then sprinkle them with cinnamon
>
> Roasted nuts
>
> Stuff some lettuce leaves with bacon, tomato slices and cream cheese
>
> Hard boiled eggs with sour cream
>
> Shrimp with low-carb chili sauce
>
> Smoked salmon and scrambled eggs
>
> Stuff a lettuce leaf with ham or turkey. You can also add mayonnaise.
>
> Greek yogurt with cinnamon

Be creative. It is easy to come up with a meal plan for a keto diet. Just be sure to use ingredients that are low in carbs, moderate in protein, and high in fat.

Simplify your breakfast

You can choose your favorite ketone breakfast like, for example, scrambled eggs, and eat it every day. If you are like some people who do not have an appetite to eat in the morning, you can just drink a hot cup of coffee or intake nothing. This will not only save you time and money but will also raise your ketone levels more quickly.

Simplify your lunch

Although dinner is the last meal of the day, you can use the opportunity of preparing your dinner to also ready your lunch for the next day. This is a good way to save on time and effort. Instead of cooking just one serving for dinner, make it two, and then keep the extra serving in the fridge for lunch the next day. And, voila, you do not have to cook again for lunch the next day.

Chapter 5: Myths

There are a number of scary myths that surround the ketogenic diet which prevent people from experiencing its benefits. You should not let fear stop you from enjoying a healthy diet, such as the keto diet. Let us separate the myths from the facts.

A healthy body needs a good amount of carbs.

Although carbohydrates are an excellent source of energy, carbs are not the only source of energy. Here is a fact as stated in a standard resource used by those in the dietetic profession: "The lower limit of dietary carbohydrate compatible with life apparently is zero, provided that adequate amounts of protein and fat are consumed."

The brain needs glucose from carbohydrate foods to function.

It is true that the brain uses the glucose found in carbohydrate foods in order to function. However, the lack of carbs does not mean that the brain can no longer function because a state of ketosis creates a glucose sparing effect. Moreover, once the body has adjusted to the ketone diet, the brain starts to fuel itself with ketones. Therefore, such myth is only true if there were no ketones in the body.

Ketosis is dangerous.

Too much of anything can be danagerous. However, when speaking of ketosis, it is important to understand the difference between ketosis and ketoacidosis. Ketosis is not dangerous, but ketoacidosis is very dangerous. There is a big difference between the two. And, as already discussed, the ketone diet does not encourage or include a state of ketoacidosis.

The ketone diet will damage your kidneys.

This scary myth arises based on a misunderstanding. Such damage to the kidneys can be caused if you consume too much protein. However, it should be noted that the keto diet is a diet that is high in fat, and not high in protein. Also, studies reveal that eating a bit more protein than is necessary does not harm the kidneys or any other parts of the body.

The keto diet, being a high-fat diet, will clog your arteries.

Since those who are on a keto diet consume foods that are high in fat, people think that this kind of eating habit will soon clog the arteries and will lead to various heart diseases. Take note that the keto diet does not allow eating any kind of fat. What it allows is only the consumption of healthy fats with good cholesterol. It is also worth remembering that cholesterol is not necessarily bad. In fact, every cell of the body also needs cholesterol.

A keto diet is not good for the colon.

Wrong. The ketone diet includes foods that are high in fiber, such as spinach and cabbage, among many others. Therefore, it is good for the colon. In fact, those who engage in a ketone diet enjoy a healthier colon, because they get to experience eating fibrous vegetables on a regular basis. This is very common on a keto diet.

The ketogenic diet will cause your muscles to shrink.

This myth can only be true if ketones are not available. Also, it must also be noted that the keto diet encourages that you eat a moderate amount of protein on a daily basis.

The keto diet will make your body weak.

One of the notable benefits of the keto diet is having improved physical and mental performance. As such, this myth is devoid of any truth. Although the body may feel weak when you first start out on a keto diet, the body will soon experience high energy levels once the body releases ketones.

Chapter 6: Common Mistakes

Those who are new to the keto diet often face the same hardships and, unfortunately, commit the same mistakes again and again. If you are about to set out on a ketogenic diet, be sure you know these common pitfalls that newbies usually encounter.

Eating processed foods

The ketogenic diet is an all-natural, whole, and real diet. Avoid pre-made Quest and Atkins bars, and focus on eating meals made from the freshest ingredients. This does not mean that you cannot eat any processed food, but be sure to keep them to a minimum. Processed foods also tend to have lots of hidden sugars, so be careful.

Wrong understanding of cholesterol

Since the keto diet is a diet that is high in fat, many people fear the sudden increase that it can make to their cholesterol level. Yes, you can expect your cholesterol level to spike up. But, you must understand that having high cholesterol is not a bad thing as long as it is the good cholesterol that is increased. In fact, the cells in your body need cholesterol.

Being impatient

Do not go for a ketogenic diet if you want to see dramatic weight loss improvements within a few days. A true keto diet is a change of lifestyle. If you just want to lose weight very quickly, then fasting or starving yourself might be the better (yet unhealthy) choice. It takes time to enjoy the maximum benefits of a keto diet. Not to mention, you first have to enter the state of ketosis, which can take about 2-3 days or more.

Not committed

Nobody says that the ketogenic diet is easy. The best diet programs in the world do not come without hardships and challenges. In order to create a meaningful change, you must make some sacrifices. Most dieters who are not fully committed to this diet fail to reach ketosis and usually give up on the first or second day. Do not be like them. When you start on a keto diet, be sure that you put your heart into it.

Eating "on time"

The ketone diet will change your eating habits. Generally, the less you eat, the better. Many dieters eat based on time demand. Meaning, they eat simply because it is morning and they think that they should have breakfast. When afternoon comes in, they eat again just because they believe that skipping lunch is not a good idea. Wrong. The ketone diet teaches that you only eat when you want to eat, and not because the clock says that it is time for you to eat. In fact, many ketone dieters skip breakfast, because they realize that they could skip breakfast without feeling uncomfortable. Unlike fasting, the ketogenic diet allows you to eat. But, only eat when you need to, or when you are really hungry.

Comparing yourself with others

Each of us are individual beings and our bodies perform generally in the same manner. But, we have individual differences.As a result, we should not engage in comparing our results or body's performance to that of others. Their performance with their chosen diet will not change or even affect your own. Focus on yourself and your diet. Another's progress or failure will not make yours any better. Learn to appreciate what you are blessed with and make ways to improve it.

Vitamins and minerals can become depleted

Although the keto diet is very much different from fasting, many people still confuse the two. Again, your keto diet should be able to sustain your body for a long term. Therefore, you must charge your body with the right and enough amounts of nutrients on a regular basis. Also, do not underestimate the magical mixture of salt and water. Salt is a source of electrolytes. Therefore, you need it when you go on a ketogenic diet. Many are concerned that consuming salt is not good for an inflamed body. But, the point is, those who are properly on a ketogenic diet do not have an inflamed body. Therefore, it is safe for you to consume salt. Of course, you should be mindful of the amount of salt that you take. The suggested amount is at least 2 teaspoons of salt daily. Also, be sure to supply your body with enough potassium, Vitamins C and D, calcium, magnesium, and others.

Not giving enough time for the body to adapt

It will take time for the body to adapt. But, once the body adapts to the keto diet, things will be much easier. Unfortunately, many dieters give up immediately when they experience the inevitable discomfort of switching to a healthy diet. Yes, you will encounter some discomfort and hardships. In fact, before you even begin a keto diet, you should already accept and prepare yourself to face some uneasiness and discomfort. The body needs time to adjust. If things get too tough for you, just think about the enormous benefits that you can reap if only you would give your body a chance to adjust to the ketogenic diet.

Consuming the wrong fats

Although the keto diet is a high-fat diet, it does not mean that you can just eat any fatty foods out there. Only choose those that have healthy fats, such as olive oil, nuts, fish oil, avocado, and others.

Not eating enough

Many dieters fail to continue their diet because of too much hunger. It is hard to deal with hunger. It is uncomfortable and can easily cause irritation. Unfortunately, many people who are on a keto diet do not eat enough, and more specifically, not enough fats. Remember that the keto diet is a diet that is high in fat. As long as you limit yourself to healthy, keto fats then you are on the right track. Another advantage of eating fats is that fats are satiating, and are effective in removing that uneasy feeling of being hungry.

Making all the changes at once

It can be shocking for the body to suddenly experience the whole, strict keto diet program at once. It is of no difference to telling someone who is used to a low carb diet to start eating tons of carbs. Therefore, it helps to prepare your body for a ketone diet by gradually decreasing the amount of carbs that you eat in a day. If you do not like foods that are high in fat, it is also a good time to start learning to appreciate such kind of food.

Chapter 7: Tips for Success

The ketogenic diet is not an easy challenge. Not only your body, but also your willpower, discipline, and self-control will be tested. Do not be discouraged if you fail to reach ketosis on your first attempt. Remember: Do not be afraid to try again.

Here are some tips that can help you succeed.

Keep a journal, avoid negative thoughts, set SMART goals, track your weight, and keep a journal.

Keep a journal

It is well advised to keep a journal. In fact, it would be helpful to start a journal even before you begin your ketone diet. Do not worry; you do not need to be a professional writer. All you need is to be open and honest so that all the records in your journal will not have any bias and clearly reflect the situation. As much as possible, your journal should have a record of everything that is related to your diet. This includes your meal plans, exercise program, diet goals, even your thoughts while engaged in the keto diet, among others.

Your journal can also function as a personal diary where you can write down your thoughts whenever you feel like giving up on the diet, as well as happy thoughts like when you first reach the state of ketosis.

Tips for tracking what you eat and drink:

Make your notes immediately after eating a meal or snack

Practice measuring or weighing your favorite foods and beverages. Become familiar with nutritional labels and serving sizes.

Rate your hunger before and after you eat using a scale of 1-10. If you eat regularly when you are not hungry, you may find that you are eating based on certain emotions or behaviors.

It may be helpful to record your thoughts, especially around meals.

Before starting a keto diet, it is wise to write in your journal how you feel when you do not follow good healthy eating habits. Write down why you want to do a ketogenic diet, your goals, as well as the importance of this diet to you. Make sure to keep these writings, because you can use them sooner or later. Somewhere along the way, a dieter usually encounters a strong temptation to give up and just return to his normal, unhealthy eating habits. If you ever find yourself in such situation, read your journal. It can give you an additional boost of inspiration to stay strong and continue with your ketone diet.

Avoid negative thoughts

Do not entertain negative thoughts such as giving up on your diet. When it comes to these matters, avoid having a dialogue with yourself. Stick to your decision and stay inspired. Also, avoid entertaining the thought of just starting over again next week or next month. Again, when you find these tempting thoughts had to ignore or resist, open your journal and read what you wrote before starting out on the keto diet. In case you were not able to make a journal before you started your ketone diet, then it is time for you to write your reasons, feelings, and diet goals, in your journal.

Tips for keeping emotional eating under control

Pause before your eat and identify your emotions

Practice conscious eating and identify your triggers for mindless eating

Maintain your food journal

Commit ant stick to a schedule

Identify ways alternative ways to cope rather than eating

Show yourself some compassion when you het a rough spot

Set aside some "me time" each day

Set SMART Goals

Though you may have huge great loss plans. We must remember that the weight was not put on overnight. Therefore, it will not go away overnight. Rapid weight loss has the tendency to backfire. A reasonable goal is starting with 10 percent. Research has shown that losing just 5-10 percent of your body weight can dramatically improve your health, boost your energy, reduce aches and pains, and decrease risks of hight blood pressure and heart disease.

SMART goals are Specific, Measurable, Achievable, Realistic, and Timed.

Be **Specific**.

Do you know what you want to achieve and why. *I want to lose 15 pounds so that my clothes fit properly.*

Is your goal **Measureable**?

Document where are you starting and track your progress.

Track your weight by weighing according to a schedule.

Tips for weighing:

Set a weight in schedule and stick to it:

Same day of week

Weigh first thing in the morning using the same set of scales

Make sure your scales are accurate and calibrated

Record your weight in a consistent place if your scales do not have memory

Do not fret over a single weight

Is your goal **Achievable**?

Chart a path to achieving your goal.

Be **Realistic**?

Make sure you are not asking too much of your self.

Schedule a **Timed** Reassessment

Set an end point to reassess and reevaluate your success.

Stay strong

Let us admit it; the keto diet is not easy. If it were so, then most people would have been physically fit. Especially in the initial stages, when hunger kicks in and you feel the temporary weakening of the body, you will be strongly tempted to just give up or simply do it again some other time. This is expected, and this is the moment when you need to be strong. Being healthy is a choice, and this is the time when you need to cling to your decision to be healthy. Prove your commitment and stay strong. Remember that once your body has adjusted to the ketone diet, things will be much easier and you can enjoy a healthy body that functions as a true fat-burning machine. Always remember: Stay strong.

Live your life

Many people who go on a low-carb diet wear a sad and miserable face. Do not be like them. Unlike fasting, the ketone diet is not about starving yourself. Rather, it is about being healthy, and healthiness is something to be enjoyed. Stop focusing on your desire to eat more or on your hunger, if any. Instead, focus on other more important things and enjoy life. This is also a good way to lessen the challenges that come with the keto diet. By focusing on other important things, you can barely feel your hunger or how the body adjusts to your new and healthy diet.

Get inspired

Inspiration can help you face the challenges that you will surely face when you go on a keto diet. Being inspired can come from many ways: You can read more about keto diet and stories of people who have succeeded. You can also make friends online with people who are currently trying the keto diet. Another good way to get a boost is to invite a friend or loved to join you in your diet. When choosing a partner, make sure to choose someone who also displays the same commitment; otherwise, he might just be a source of discouragement instead of inspiration.

Building an environment to succeed is also very important. Take the time to modify your surrounding to ensure that you are successful. Your surroundings can go a long way to support your weight loss efforts. Be sure to assess what items in your home, at work, or even in your car that need to be removed and what needs to be added. First and foremost, rid the kitchen of unhealthy foods and replace them with foods that fall within your diet plan. Chances are if you do not have those items to avoid within reach, you will not make the effort to go and get them. Acknowledge that preparation is key. Make sure that you prepare your lunch and have snacks on hand during the day. Remember that this is your weight loss journey and you are in control of your success. When ordering in or going out to eat, your coworkers are not considering your special dietary requirements. It is not their responsibility, it is yours.

Pray

Prayer works. What better way to face the challenges of a ketone diet than receiving spiritual guidance and empowerment from the Almighty? Therefore, pray — pray for the strength to succeed. And even if you are not a spiritual person, studies show that praying, even just for the sake of doing something, has beneficial psychological effects.

Stay motivated

How motivated you are is an important element of success. Usually, dieters are highly motivated at the start of a ketone diet. However, once hunger starts to kick in, their motivation also begins to wane. And the more they experience this hunger, the more they lose their motivation to continue with the diet. Although this is normal, this is not the right state of mind to be in. A good way to keep your motivation strong is by reading the reasons why you have decided to pursue a ketone diet in the first place. Again, having a journal is what makes this possible. Another way to stay motivated is by appreciating any improvements that you have already had, if any. You can also read success stories and testimonials of other ketone dieters. However, sometimes, you simply have to accept that nothing can seem to motivate you enough, and the only way to move forward with the diet is to force yourself to stay strong and continue to hold on. As such, having a strong willpower would be of great use.

Get Moving

Exercising and increasing your activity level can cause you to regain energy and vitality while losing weight.

Exercise has several benefits. e cannot list them all here but, it is worth noting that when compared to those with a sedentary live stile, active folks are less likely to develop heart disease, high blood pressure, diabetes, colon cancer, breast cancer, dementia, depression, back pain, and osteoporosis. Those who exercise report better sleep patterns few colds, and less stress than those who do not exercise.

While dietary changes seem to be the key to losing weight, exercise is also helpful and it is critical for keeping the unwanted pounds off.

Tips for sitting less each day:

Stand or walk while talking on the phone

Take standing breaks every 15 to 20 minutes throughout the day

Take a walk before or after eating lunch

Walk down the hall to talk with colleagues instead of sending emails

Replace a coffee break with a 10 minute walk

NOTE: Always check with your healthcare provider before starting a physical activity program or increasing the intensity of your current program. Consult with your healthcare provider about dietary changes and exercise that is best for your and your personal condition.

Conclusion

Thank for making it through to the end of this book, let's hope it was informative and able to provide you with all of the tools you need to achieve your goals whatever they may be.

The next step is to apply everything that you have learned. Begin your ketogenic diet, and enjoy the wonderful benefits that it offers. Best wishes!

Finally, if you found this book useful in any way, a positive review on Amazon is always appreciated!

Description

The *Ketogenic Diet* is your one-stop guide to everything you need to know about the keto-eating habits. It explains the important principles and provides detailed guidelines on what you should do in order to see results while on this diet. This book is the best ketogenic diet manual for beginners.

Learn:

- What is a ketogenic diet?

- The foods you should eat and those that you should avoid

- What is ketosis?

- The common pitfalls to avoid while on the ketogenic diet

- Common myths of the ketogenic diet

- Some common side effects of the keto diet and how to prevent or avoid them

- How to turn your body into a fat burning machine

- And more!